EASY HEALTHCARE:

BEFORE YOU GET SICK

By

Lori-Ann Rickard

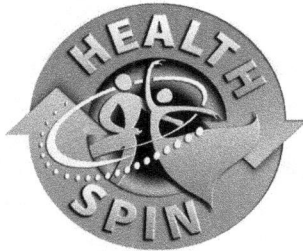

Presented by
Expert Health Press

For Alyssa and Cassie,
you are the lights of my life.

TABLE OF CONTENTS

INTRODUCTION

At some point, everyone who's been sick or had an ill loved one has had to ask the inevitable question: should you go to an **urgent care facility** or an emergency room to seek care?

In order to determine the answer, you must **triage** yourself or your loved one. Triage is the word medical professionals use when they assess how serious a patient's condition is. The more critical a patient's condition, the sooner and more aggressively he or she will be treated. Applying the same principles to yourself and your loved ones is not only the best way to be a responsible patient, but it can save you time, money, and needless worry.

No Brainer—Serious Symptoms Need a Serious Response

Obviously, if you experience major trauma—you're involved in a car accident or fall off a ladder—you shouldn't hesitate to go to the emergency room. The best response to any serious situation is to immediately call 911. A serious healthcare problem would include:

- Unconsciousness
- Heavy bleeding
- Difficulty breathing
- Excessive pain
- Seizures
- Large bruise or other obvious injury
- Serious neck or back injury
- Skin suddenly becoming cold or clammy or skin color changes
- Shock
- Any other problems as directed by your doctor

When faced with any of these symptoms, you should not hesitate to call 911. Also, follow your doctor's orders if he or she has given you specific instructions to go to the emergency room if you experience certain symptoms associated with an illness, pre-existing condition, or ongoing treatment.

What If It's Not Obvious?

What if you haven't fallen off a ladder? What if you're not sure whether you have an injury or illness that requires a trip to the emergency room?

If you're not sure whether you should go to the emergency room or not, the first person you should call is your primary care doctor. This is one of most important reasons to establish a good relationship with a primary care physician. You want to select a physician who knows you and your family personally and is available when you have a question. If the practice you go to is merely a "patient mill" where you never see the same doctor twice, consider looking for a new provider. You interview babysitters and talk to car mechanics before they provide you service. Why wouldn't you do the same with a potential doctor?

Even the best physicians are not always available, though. It may seem like the one time you need to talk to him or her, you get the "dreaded" answering machine message saying the office is closed and to call 911 if "this is a true emergency."

This is why you want to take charge of your healthcare long before you are sick, injured, or confronted with the "call 911 or not" question. First know the difference between a real life-threatening emergency and a less critical situation. Second, know your own healthcare conditions and needs as well as those of your loved ones. Finally, understand how the healthcare system works and how to be a smart consumer of their services. By knowing some basic guidelines, you can avoid many unnecessary frustrations and costs for yourself or your loved one.

So what are the 7 things you need to know before getting sick?

1.

BE PROACTIVE ABOUT WHEN YOU SEEK HEALTHCARE

Most illnesses happen over time. It's rare to have a sudden need for healthcare that isn't related to an accident or traumatic injury. This is why it's important to proactively care for yourself and your loved ones. Continually monitor your health and seek out **preventative care** (e.g. regular physicals and health screenings such as mammograms or colonoscopies). Identifying an illness or condition early on is the best way to avoid a trip to the emergency room in the future.

Also, as you are getting sick, notice your symptoms. Are you familiar with them? Keep notes with dates when certain symptoms appear for certain chronic problems. If and when these symptoms repeat themselves, call the doctor's office during their open hours and ask to speak to the nurse. Triage yourself. It's important that you're able to describe in detail your specific symptoms. For example, don't say, "I feel awful" or "I've never felt so sick." Instead, specifically describe your symptoms:

I'm calling because I have a bad cold. My symptoms started on Monday with yellow discharge and I'm coughing. The coughing is keeping me up at night. I have a temperature of 101.3 and I have had that temperature for 36 hours. In the last three hours, I have thrown up three times. I appear to be throwing up green stomach liquid.

If you provide the nurse with specific details on your condition, he or she can provide much more accurate and helpful information to the doctor. Also, if the doctor needs to see you, you can still get an appointment during the week.

You should also keep loved ones informed about how you're feeling. If during the week you feel faint, it's important to let someone close to you know. If your condition worsens and you're unable to take care of yourself, it's important for those around you to be aware of your condition. For example, if you live alone and don't feel well, ask a neighbor to check in on you. Resist the urge to be a hermit because you don't feel well. Sometimes a friendly call is just what you need.

DON'T GET SICK ON THE WEEKEND (OR, CAN YOU SURVIVE UNTIL MONDAY?)

Many illnesses, serious or not, evolve slowly. A simple example everyone's lived: on Monday night, you start to feel like you're getting a cold, but, no, you have meetings, the kids' soccer practice, that dinner with that friend. By Friday night, after ignoring your symptoms all week, you feel like you want to die. Is that cold turning into something else? You call the doctor and get the answering machine.

It comes as a surprise to many people that doctors and other healthcare workers keep the same business hours we all do. And, like most businesses, staff in a doctor's office becomes scarce on Friday afternoons. As a practical matter, other than emergency care, very little healthcare is offered on the weekends.

This is true whether you're an inpatient in the hospital or you're merely seeking care as an outpatient. Doctors and nurses work on the weekend to treat people who need emergency care. They rarely see patients in their office on the weekend except for an occasional Saturday, if you're lucky. If you or your loved one is an inpatient at a hospital, you'll quickly notice that very little happens on the weekend. It's unlikely that you'll get physical therapy on the weekend and no non-emergency surgeries occur on the weekend. For the most part, you'll simply sit in the hospital until Monday morning to get anything other than basic care.

Back to our example, if you are feeling sick all week, Friday night at 9 p.m. isn't a good time to decide you need healthcare services. If you wait until Friday night, it's likely that the only healthcare services available are in urgent care or the emergency room, two options you should NOT use for a bad cold (or the sinus infection it may have become).

KNOW WHEN YOUR DOCTOR IS AVAILABLE

If you have a choice, always choose to be seen by your own doctor. Your doctor is familiar with you and your history, while an urgent care physician or emergency room doctor has no way to know your entire health history. Additionally, the urgent care doctor is only going to provide enough care to get you back to your family physician.

Having a good relationship with your family doctor and his or her office staff is very important. As you're getting sick, you want to call the office, tell them your symptoms and, if there's any doubt, make an appointment to see the doctor. Don't wait until the weekend, when your symptoms are worse, you're dehydrated, and can't talk to your doctor until Monday.

Get familiar with the schedule at your doctor's office. Most are generally open only during the week, but some may be closed one day a week, have longer hours on certain days of the week, or be open one Saturday a month. This information is important for you to know. For example, if you know that your doctor's office is closed on Fridays and you're getting sick throughout the week, you should check with your doctor early Thursday morning to determine if you need any care. By planning ahead, you will avoid having to suffer through the weekend or worst yet, sitting in an emergency room for hours only to be told that you should see your doctor on Monday.

Calling the doctor's office after hours is also less than ideal. First, the phone message at the doctor's office will always advise you to go to the emergency room. However, the reason for the message is a legal one, not a medical one. It's not that most patients calling at off hours are critically ill. Doctor's offices don't want to assume the risk of telling you to wait when something bad might happen. It's safer for the doctor to direct you to emergency room than tell you to wait for an appointment, even if in all likelihood you don't need to go. Second, doctors rotate taking off hours calls for the office, so the odds of getting a doctor who doesn't know you are high. And what will that doctor likely tell you? Go to the emergency room.

THE BOTTOM LINE...

- Monitor your health so that illnesses or conditions are diagnosed well before they become critical.

- When symptoms do appear, pay attention, and communicate them in detail to your family doctor.

- Always call your family doctor first. Know his or her work schedule.

- Remember that doctors and most healthcare providers don't work weekends. If you get sick during the work week, take care of it during the work week.

- Don't go to the emergency room just because the recorded message on the doctor's answering machine says you should.

2.

BEWARE OF URGENT CARE

If your illness comes on quickly or you're feeling too ill to wait until your doctor's office opens, you may consider going to the local urgent care clinic. Some people believe that a visit there is the same as going to their family doctor. This is simply not true.

URGENT CARE IS NOT YOUR FAMILY DOCTOR

Going to an urgent care clinic is very different than seeing your family doctor. At the urgent care clinic, staff will rarely know who you are and what your medical history might be. Likewise, you will know nothing about the urgent care doctor's credentials or specialty, nor will you have any idea how long he or she has been in practice—all important information when assessing whether or not this is a doctor who can help you.

URGENT CARE CENTERS—THE FAST FOOD OF HEALTHCARE

Often, doctors who work at urgent care clinics have "day jobs" practicing medicine somewhere else, the urgent care center being a way to make extra money. Would your family doctor moonlight at an urgent care clinic? Unlikely. Many of the doctors who work at urgent care clinics are just out of school or don't have established medical practices. While this doesn't mean that all urgent care doctors are inexperienced or substandard, it does mean that, as a patient, you will have no way of knowing how competent that doctor you see is. Is this how you want to approach a potentially important health issue?

Additionally, because many doctors moonlight at urgent care facilities, it's unlikely they will see you again. Urgent care clinic doctors are often incentivized to see patients quickly and get them out the door. We all know that certain illnesses and medical conditions can be complex and require much more than a ten-minute, first-time visit. To fully treat an issue, a physician evaluating you should know you and your medical history. That same doctor should also be available later on when complications or new symptoms occur, or if you simply have further questions. If the urgent care doctor only covers one day a week, it's unlikely he or she will be available for any sort of follow up. Urgent care clinics also have limited resources, such as x-ray machines or laboratory facilities. If your condition requires any of these services, you will likely be sent somewhere else.

Many urgent care facilities encourage their staff to prescribe medication because patients are looking for a "quick fix" by coming to the clinic. It can be difficult for the patient to hear that a midnight visit to urgent care cost $50, but the treatment for what turns out to be a bad cold is merely rest and fluids. In this situation, the urgent care doctor can feel compelled to prescribe an antibiotic when in fact it is unnecessary, or even potentially dangerous.

To that point, an urgent care facility will likely not have access to your medical history. Therefore, if you do not bring a list of all your medications, you may find that the urgent care doctor will prescribe medications that are either inappropriate given your current prescriptions or not your family doctor's medication of choice for you. For instance, if you are having a great deal of pain, the urgent care doctor may prescribe Vicodin. In the alternative, your family doctor may have prescribed the less powerful and non-habit-forming Tylenol 3 based on your previous medical history.

BEWARE OF PAYMENT ISSUES

When you or your loved one feel sick enough to visit urgent care, thinking about insurance coverage is less important than finding an open clinic close to home. But it's an important question. Because patients often assume that visiting an urgent care facility is the same as going to their family doctor, they often take for granted that it will be covered by their insurance, which is not always the case.

If you don't know in advance, call your insurance company or review your policy before visiting an urgent care clinic. When you get to the clinic, ask about coverage prior to signing forms and receiving care. Ask what the charges are. Additionally, if you will receive any testing, such as x-rays or blood work, be certain to understand the cost.

When you're sick, it's difficult to remember that you'll be responsible for any charges not covered by your insurance. Every healthcare provider gives the patient many forms to sign when they first arrive, and you'll be asked to fill them all out on your first visit to the urgent care clinic. All of those forms have significance and should be read thoroughly before signing them. One of the forms will clearly state that you're responsible for any services not covered by insurance at the time the services are rendered. Do not be overwhelmed by the amount of forms and be sure to ask any questions prior to getting services.

Finally, not only may the urgent care center not accept your insurance, it may cost more than going to see your doctor, since these facilities often charge a premium for their services. And, depending on how your insurance is structured, you may unexpectedly end up paying more out of your own pocket as a result.

URGENT CARE IS NOT A REPLACEMENT FOR THE EMERGENCY ROOM

Just like some patients believe the urgent care clinic is the same as their family doctor's office, others believe it's an emergency-room substitute. Again, that's not the case. Many health conditions can be treated without going to the emergency room; but if you have a life-threatening illness, don't waste time going to urgent care. As described above, symptoms such as loss of consciousness, chest pain, and difficulty breathing should only be treated in an emergency room where a full range of experienced specialists with advanced technology and treatments stand ready to help you.

If you are having a life-threatening emergency and make the mistake of going first to an urgent care center, the urgent care center will merely call 911 to have you transported to the nearest hospital. In this case, you'll receive the bill from the urgent care center for doing nothing more than what you or your loved ones could have done.

THE BOTTOM LINE...

- An urgent care center is not your family doctor.

- An urgent care doctor will not know your medical history.

- You will not know the skills and competency of an urgent care doctor.

- An urgent care center will not have all the same equipment and services as your doctor's office or the hospital.

- An urgent care center won't always take your health insurance.

- Urgent care centers often charge a premium for their services.

- Urgent care centers are not emergency rooms. If you're experiencing serious symptoms go the emergency room or call 911.

3.

911 IS ONLY FOR A REAL EMERGENCY

Triage 101: If you are suffering from a life-threatening illness or injury, call 911. If you suffer from any of the symptoms outlined earlier, call 911. If your doctor instructs you to call 911 if you have certain symptoms, call 911.

Below is outlined what you can expect when you make that call, but the expense and complication are of little consequence when the emergency is real. If, however, you're certain your condition is not life-threatening, making your way to the hospital in a less dramatic way can save significant time and money.

AMBULANCE CARE IS DETERMINED BY YOUR CALL

There are three different types of ambulances: basic life support, advanced life support, and critical care. You should understand that the type of ambulance sent will be determined by the statements you make when you call. So, it's important that, if at all possible, the person making the call can calmly inform the dispatcher where you are located and what the symptoms are. The caller will then need to stay on the phone while the dispatcher contacts the ambulance company, which will send out the ambulance with the equipment appropriate to your emergency.

If you're the one needing transport, someone should follow the ambulance to the hospital or you should instruct the technicians to contact a loved one, if at all possible. You will need an advocate when you arrive at the hospital. No one should go to the emergency room alone.

AMBULANCE WILL TAKE YOU TO THE CLOSEST HOSPITAL

Ambulances are generally required to take you to the hospital closest to where your emergency occurred. This doesn't mean you'll be taken to a hospital of your choice or one that is best suited to treat you. Even if the closest hospital is one with a poor reputation, the ambulance company will still have to take you there. In a real emergency, time is of the essence. This is one of the many reasons why you should not call an ambulance unless you need one. By taking your own transportation, the choice of hospitals is under your control.

AMBULANCE TRANSPORTATION IS EXPENSIVE

An ambulance ride is very expensive, and, depending on your insurance it may or may not be covered by your policy. If you don't have a life-threatening illness or are not experiencing the symptoms described above, consider whether or not you want to call an ambulance. Some people call ambulance companies not because they need emergency care, but because they simply don't feel well and need a way to the hospital. After they get the bill, they regret not finding some other way to get to there.

GET OTHER TRANSPORTATION

Consider whether you have an alternate means of transportation. Can a loved one drive you to the hospital? Can a neighbor drive you? Are you well enough to drive yourself? Depending on your circumstances, a family member may be able to get you to the emergency room quicker than an ambulance.

AVOID AIR AMBULANCE TRIPS

As healthcare evolves, hospitals continue to look for ways to attract and keep patients within their service system. One of the ways the hospital does this is to have an air ambulance helicopter. In an urban area, this is silly. An ambulance with "lights and sirens" can usually get to the nearest hospital quicker than a helicopter. As you can imagine, air ambulance transportation is very expensive, much more so than a regular ambulance ride. Unless you're in a rural set-ting where you need a large hospital to care for you that is far away, you should avoid using a helicopter if other options are available. If you would just like to ride in a helicopter because it's cool, wait until you're feeling better and take a ride for fun.

BE PREPARED FOR A HOSPITAL STAY

If you do call an ambulance, you or your loved one should pack a bag with all the things you may want at the hospital. For an older patient who may get cold, you might want to bring a warm blanket or jacket since they may have to wait a long time. Also, don't take any valuables with you to the hospital. Leave your precious watches, rings, and other valuables at home. Things can have a way of disap-pearing as you're being taken from place to place within a hospital. It's better to leave all of your important items at home.

Additionally, always take your Medical Life List as well as your insurance card and your driver's license (or other form of identifi-cation). This information is important to have readily available for both the ambulance and the hospital.

THE BOTTOM LINE...

- The level of ambulance care is determined by your call. The more serious your condition, the more sophisticated the equipment will be on the vehicle.

- If possible have someone come with you or follow the ambulance to the hospital.

- Ambulances must take you to the hospital closest to where the emergency occurred, not to the hospital of your choice.

- Ambulance transportation is extremely expensive and not always covered by health insurance.

- Don't call an ambulance if you have another way to get to the hospital and aren't experiencing serious symptoms.

- Ambulances are not "hospital taxis" and should not be treated as such.

- Avoid air ambulance trips.

- Be prepared to stay in the hospital. Take your ID and your Medical Life List with you.

4.

WHAT TO EXPECT IN THE EMERGENCY ROOM

If you have gone by ambulance to the emergency room or have decided that the emergency room is your only option, you should be prepared for what to expect. For a life-threatening illness or accident, the emergency room is absolutely the best place to be. Most hospitals have the staff and facilities necessary to manage most life-threatening situations in the most effective and efficient manner possible. In a life-threatening emergency, minutes matter. However, if you do not have a life-threatening illness, the emergency room will certainly have some drawbacks.

CHOOSE WISELY

As already described, if you go by ambulance to the hospital, the ambulance will take you to the closest facility, not necessarily the best facility. Therefore, if you want to choose which hospital you'll be treated in, you want to use your own transportation. Many people assume that every hospital is the same. This is simply not true.

Hospitals are focusing more on customer service and the "patient experience" as they compete for your healthcare dollars. Some present themselves like high-end resorts, with glossy advertisements, impressive lobbies, and waiting rooms with wi-fi and flat screen televisions. But remember, you aren't looking for a great "hotel" to stay at for a few days. You are choosing a hospital that will impact your life or that of your loved one. What's important is the competency of doctors and nurses who care for the patients and the effectiveness of the hospital administration. Every hospital has great healthcare providers working in them; however, what is the overall reputation of the hospital? You can easily ask for references from your primary care doctor or do some research on the internet. It won't take long for you to determine what hospitals have great ratings and what hospitals don't.

Location also should be one of the factors you consider. For example, if one of your children will be in the hospital for some time, it will be much easier for you to care for your other children at home if the hospital is located nearby. However, this is only one factor, and not always the most important. No matter how close the hospital is, you'll likely be at the hospital most of the time and will need to find family and friends who can help you care for your other children. If the local children's hospital is the best choice for your child's illness, then driving another ten minutes to get there should not be the determining factor.

You should also be aware of what services hospitals in your area offer and which hospitals your doctors practice at. We all know of hospitals that don't provide a full complement of care. For example, the hospital closest to you may be a small, local one that does not have the specialized services you need. Additionally, most doctors only work at certain hospitals. For example, if your doctor is employed by a hospital system, it's the only one where he or she will have credentials. So, you shouldn't expect to see your primary care physician no matter what hospital you select. If you do go to a hospital where your doctor is not **credentialed**, you will be assigned an unknown primary care physician who is.

THE ER DOES NOT KNOW YOU

One of the most important factors in receiving good medical treatment is knowledge of your health history. How a healthcare professional approaches various symptoms is partially based on what he or she knows about the illnesses or conditions you have and the results of recent tests. If the healthcare provider knows nothing about you, he or she will need to start from scratch. Although health information technology is developing, the healthcare industry has not yet evolved to the point where someone can access your health history from any location. This is the primary reason why it's so important for you to keep an updated record that contains all of your important health history, including any surgeries, medications, allergies, and procedures. Even if you have that complete list, it's likely that the emergency room doctor will want to repeat various tests or procedures, for which you will be charged.

Also, it's very unlikely that your primary care doctor will come to the emergency room to see you. If you are in a hospital where your primary care doctor is credentialed, he or she will see you once are admitted to the hospital. However, if your primary care doctor does not work at the hospital you have chosen, doctors whom you do not know will see you.

This is one of the reasons that, as I cared for my aging parents, I insisted on selecting doctors who worked out of one health system. We live in an urban area so there were a lot of choices. I chose doctors who worked at a health system with a good reputation that was also close by our homes. By choosing doctors who could all access the same records, I no longer needed to run to different healthcare providers for documentation every time my dad was in need of hospital care.

Also, having healthcare providers who know you is especially important as you age. Although unfortunate, many seniors get taken to the emergency room with no support system, and it's easy for a busy doctor there to dismiss a senior's symptoms as simply the result of "being old." In the case of my father, he was mentally competent but could appear to have a form of dementia due to an unrelated health condition. If we had gone to an emergency room or hospital where his records weren't available or he was alone, it would have been likely that the doctors would have not looked beyond age as the cause for any change in mental capacity.

EMERGENCY ROOM DOCTORS ARE FOR EMERGENCIES

You should know that emergency room doctors are there to treat true emergencies. If your situation is not an emergency, they won't see you until after they've treated more critical patients. These doctors are backed up by a team of specialists who are "**on call**" to come into the emergency room if needed. So, in the case of a serious accident or life-threatening illness, these specialists will be immediately available. Not so if your condition is not serious. Even if you're feeling terrible with a non-urgent flu virus, it's highly unlikely that a doctor is going to come to the emergency room in the middle of the night or on a weekend to see you. What will happen is that, after a long wait, the emergency room doctor will either send you to your primary care doctor when his or her office opens or provide you with some limited care until that time. Moreover, the bill for this will be generally very expensive, and you'll be expected to pay even if it was only to be sent to your primary care doctor.

THE "WAIT" FROM HELL

If you choose to go to the emergency room and you do not have a life-threatening illness, it's likely that you'll wait a very long time to receive care. Because the emergency room is equipped to handle life-threatening illnesses as quickly as possible, the emergency room must triage each patient to determine if he or she needs immediate care. Because there is no way for the emergency room to determine how many patients they'll have at any given time, they must see the sickest patients first. Therefore, even though you aren't feeling well, you may have to wait a very long time to receive the various tests and exams that you need before someone can treat you.

For example, if you're an elderly patient who fell and needs an x-ray, you will not be seen when you first arrive in the emergency room. The emergency room must first attend to those who arrive from car accidents, house fires, and shootings. Many of these events occur during the evening hours or on weekends. If you happen to arrive Friday at 8:30 pm and a serious car accident occurred at 8 pm, it's likely that the hospital will be focused on the individuals involved in the car accident for quite some time. It is not unusual to spend more than twenty-four hours in an emergency room waiting for a specific doctor or a test to determine what care to provide. Waiting a long period of time in a cold, sterile emergency room isn't easy when you don't feel well.

For example, my eighty-five-year-old father fell and broke his hip on a Sunday. Although he was in a great deal of pain from what we thought might be a fractured hip, he was otherwise fine. First, we called his primary care doctor to get his advice. As a result, rather than taking a trip to the emergency room and waiting twelve hours for an x-ray that his doctor was unlikely to use, we chose to wait until Monday morning to go to see the orthopedic surgeon. That morning, we went to the office, determined that his hip was fractured, and scheduled him for surgery. For a very independent, proud man, it was much more comfortable for him to be in his house with family on Sunday evening rather than in a cold emergency room where very little care would be provided. This is simply one example of being responsible for your own healthcare needs and making a rational determination regarding what care is necessary and what's truly an emergency.

Additionally, another important piece of information to know is that everything moves slower at a hospital in the evenings and on weekends. There is less staff available, generally, in the emergency room for tests such as x-rays or MRIs. Further, if your illness can wait, the emergency room will likely conduct the tests you need, but send you to see a specialist Monday morning. Often, that specialist will want different tests, and you will be charged for both sets of tests.

BEWARE OF OBSERVATION CHARGES

Most people believe that once you enter a hospital you are "admitted" to the hospital. In most cases, this assumption makes sense because you're physically in the hospital when you go to the emergency room. However, you should know that being in the emergency room does not mean you're "admitted" to the hospital. This is very important to understand because your insurance may not cover some of your care if you are not admitted.

Many emergency rooms have a designation called "**observation**." If you are deemed to be in observation, your insurance will treat you as an outpatient. For many people, especially seniors, this designation can be very expensive. Under **Medicare**, there is a limit on how much the hospital will be paid for outpatient services. You could be getting the same care after being admitted to the hospital and Medicare would cover the services.

So what is observation? Observation is a status determined by the hospital that means you are too sick to go home but not sick enough to be admitted to the hospital. Observation status requires a doctor's order, and you could be in the emergency room in observation for several days. The hospital may be running several tests in order to determine whether you should go home or be "admitted" to the hospital. Medicare guidelines suggest that "observation" should be limited to twenty-four to forty-eight hours. However, many hospitals hold patients in observation status for several days.

Because Medicare considers observation to be an outpatient service, the senior will have to pay a **co-pay** and **deductible** for the doctor's fees. Additionally, he or she will have to pay hospital charges for any routine medications they currently take if they are prescribed while in observation.

Further, it is very important to understand that a Medicare patient in observation will not have coverage for nursing care or rehabilitation even though a doctor may order it. Such care generally needs to be preceded by a hospital admission. In order to be eligible for nursing care or rehabilitation, the Medicare patient must have spent three consecutive days (midnight to midnight) admitted to the hospital, not including the day of discharge.

Medicare does not require hospitals to inform patients when they are in observation status. The only way to know is to ask. Medicare patients also often believe they've been admitted when in fact they have not. Your doctor may even agree that you need to be admitted, but the decision is ultimately made by the hospital. So, it's important to be proactive, which can be difficult when you aren't feeling well. This is another reason why you must bring someone with you when you go to the hospital to act as your advocate, asking questions and finding out the answers.

Most hospitals have a patient advocate office or ombudsman office. If you aren't getting the answers you need, you should ask to speak with someone who is available to assist patients with getting the answers they need. Remember, waiting to find out your status until you are discharged from the hospital is too late. If you're a Medicare patient there are ways to appeal your bill once it is received; however, it's much more difficult to get the decision changed after the fact.

THE BOTTOM LINE...

- When the ambulance takes you to the nearest hospital, it's not always the best hospital for your illness.

- Before you ever need to go, determine which hospitals in your area are best for you.

- If you aren't experiencing a real emergency, be prepared to fall to the bottom of the list for treatment in an emergency room.

- Don't expect to see a specialist or your own primary care doctor in the emergency room if you aren't experiencing serious symptoms.

- Expect long waits in the emergency room if your condition isn't serious.

- Expect even longer waits at night or on weekends.

- Be sure that your trip to the emergency room is covered by your insurance if your condition isn't critical.

- Be aware that hospitals can designate you as in observation and not admitted, which may be very costly.

5.

ALWAYS HAVE YOUR MEDICAL LIFE LIST

Because you never know when you might need urgent healthcare or see a doctor you don't know, it's important to keep with you a copy of all important health information for you and your loved ones, something we call your Medical Life List. When you're sick or have a family member who needs immediate medical attention, you rarely have the time or the resources to gather your health information.

A Medical Life List should include your personal information such as name, address, social security number, driver's license number, and employer information. Next, the list should detail all of your healthcare providers' information, such as their names, addresses, specialties, and hospital affiliation. Next, you should include any information about major health events, including any hospitalizations and changes in insurance. Also, for children, you should keep track of illnesses, vaccinations, and days of missed school.

Remember when you or your loved one adds or changes a doctor or medication; simply add it to your Medical Life List or that of your loved one. Place the date of the update on the list. This way you'll always know that you have the most recent list. Always remember to keep the list in a secure format and shred any old copies. If you're comfortable with computers and can keep a digitally encrypted copy of the list, only keep an electronic copy of the list. However, if you prefer to keep a paper copy, do so. You should also have the list readily available in case of an emergency. It should be easily accessible if you have to ask someone else to assist with your healthcare.

You should also keep copies of important medical records, tests, and laboratory results. Having this information readily available is important to receive quick and efficient healthcare.

The Bottom Line...

- Maintain a Medical Life List: an updated list of your medical history and that of your loved ones.

- As your health history changes, make sure you update the list.

- Keep the list in a secure place.

- Know where the list is at all times and make sure your loved ones know where your list is should you experience an emergency.

- If you or your loved one is going to the ER, make sure that you have the list with you.

- Also keep copies of important medical records, tests, and laboratory results.

6.

BE PREPARED TO BE ADMITTED TO THE HOSPITAL

If you choose to go to the emergency room with a non-emergency problem, it's likely that you will be discharged with instructions to see your family doctor. However, the emergency room doctor may decide to admit you to the hospital.

TRANSFERRING TO A DIFFERENT HOSPITAL IS RARELY AN OPTION

Once you have been seen in one hospital's emergency room, it's very difficult to be transferred to a different hospital. When an emergency room doctor treats you, he or she is in charge of your care. In almost all circumstances, that doctor will want to admit you to either the hospital you are at or, if you need a higher level of care, to a larger hospital affiliated with their emergency room.

If you believe that you or your loved one is at the wrong hospital, you should immediately start the transfer process. In order to be transferred, you will need a doctor's order, but you should know that doctors are very hesitant to agree to a transfer simply due to a patient's personal preference. In some cases you will be transferred no matter what your preference. Certain types of insurance require that when a patient is admitted to an out-of-network hospital, he or she must be transferred when stable to a facility that is covered by that insurance plan. This may take some time and you may have to pay out-of-pocket for some of the costs. This is why it is simply better to go to the right hospital in the first place.

If you have chosen the correct hospital and emergency room, you want to begin to think about what you need during your hospital stay.

ASK YOUR PRIMARY CARE PHYSICIAN FOR RECOMMENDATIONS

One in the hospital, you or your loved ones will first likely want to contact your primary care physician for recommendations regarding a specialist for your illness or condition. For instance, if you have broken a hip, you will need an orthopedic surgeon who specializes in hips. If you don't have the name of an orthopedic surgeon of your own, the hospital will likely assign you to one out of their rotation. Obviously, if your primary care physician works regularly at the hospital, he or she may be able to recommend an orthopedic surgeon.

This is another reason why you want to be at a hospital where your primary care physician is credentialed. Being at a hospital where your doctor does not practice means you will be seen by both primary care physicians and specialists who do not know you or know anything about your health history. It's not necessarily the best plan to be operated on by the specialist who was just "on call" that evening or simply next on the hospital list for referrals. You may get a specialist who is superb or you may get a specialist who no one would recommend.

PICK ONE DOCTOR TO BE IN CHARGE OF YOUR CARE

You're likely to have many different doctors seeing you while you're in the hospital. If you're having your hip replaced, but you also have heart issues, your cardiologist is likely to also see you or consult on your case while you're in the hospital. If you also have problems with your kidneys, a nephrologist may also see you. It's very important that you have one specialist who is in charge of your overall care. That doctor needs to coordinate all the other doctors. Coordination of care is very difficult since all the doctors see you at different times during the day. You should make sure you discuss with the "in charge" doctor your expectation that he or she will manage your "team" of doctors. If you don't believe all your doctors understand who is in charge of coordinating your care, you should ask for a meeting with the doctors to discuss any issues.

WHAT TYPE OF ROOM DO YOU WANT?

Healthcare is changing every day, with hospitals competing more and more for patients, and becoming more customer focused as a result. Many hospitals now offer private rooms or semi-private rooms. Depending on your needs and your insurance coverage, you may want to ask for a private room. In a semi-private room, you will likely have a roommate. With a roommate you will have to be present for all of his or her care and possibly be woken up in the middle of the night as a result. Additionally, every time your roommate has a visitor you will have to listen to their conversation, and those visitors may be with them throughout the day and possibly most of the night. Conversely, your roommate may not want you to have extensive visitors since they may disturb him or her. Constant television viewing, differing views on religion or politics, a roommate's need for small talk are other factors that make it difficult to get the rest you need when sharing a room.

All of these things should be considered when you ask about the cost of a private room, which, of course, is more expensive and may not be covered by your insurance. Because patients often want private rooms, some areas of the hospital or the entire hospital may have private rooms. If this is important to you, you should inquire about where in the hospital you are going to be located and what types of rooms are available there.

HAVE SOMEONE WITH YOU WHENEVER POSSIBLE

Some people believe that when their loved one is in the hospital, staff is with them twenty-four hours a day. Although hospitals provide care around the clock, the nurses and doctors have many patients to care for. Due to cost cutting and various other changes in healthcare, it's becoming more and more difficult for the nurses and doctors to attend to every patient's needs. This is one of the reasons why you should have someone with you at all times, if possible, to act as your advocate and take care of the small things you need. A family member, close friend or a combination of both can be essential to receiving the care you need. Even if you cannot have somebody with you at all times, it's important to have somebody with you as often as possible, especially when you see the doctor. When you're sick, it's not the best time to attempt to coordinate your care on your own or keep track of the many details associated with your hospital stay.

TAKE NOTES

If possible, you should have someone taking notes about who comes and goes from your hospital room. There are many different healthcare providers who will visit your room and you should know who those individuals are, what their specialties are, and how they think you're doing each day. A hospital day is a very long for a patient. It can be very difficult to remember when people come and go, whether you have gotten the results of the various tests being run, and what the prognosis is for your stay.

A hospital employs many different healthcare providers. Although somebody may walk into your room who appears to be a doctor, he or she may simply be a medical student in training. Hospital training programs dictate that interns and residents come to your room first. An **intern** is still in medical school, while a **resident** has graduated from medical school and is being trained in his or her specialty. The interns and residents gather all the data regarding your status and report it to the doctor in charge of your care.

It's important for you to understand who these people are since you'll be more interested in your own doctor's opinion than in their opinions. If you attempt to get the opinion of every intern and resident, you'll rapidly become confused about your care. Your doctor will ultimately decide how to proceed with your care and may not listen to the opinions of the intern or resident. Indeed, it's easy to focus on the opinions of the intern or resident since he or she is likely to take more time with you, while your doctor is busy trying to get his or her hospital rounds done each day.

Once your doctor visits, you'll often need to stop him or her to ask your questions. Some attending doctors will actually stand in the doorway of the room to discuss your care. That way, they can see patients quickly. If this happens and you have questions, simply ask them to come into the room. The doctor may say that he or she is busy and will come back later. While you need to be sensitive to the fact that your doctor has many responsibilities, getting answers to your questions is part of caring for you. Since the attending doctor will be billing every day he sees you in the hospital, you are entitled to answers to your questions. You may also want to write down your questions (or have your loved one do so) in advance of seeing the doctor.

If you're in the hospital for surgery, you may be visited not only by your surgeon but also by another surgeon from his group or practice who will check your status on his or her behalf. Keeping track of names will help you to determine whom you need to talk to if you have a question or concern. A simple way to do this is to merely ask for the doctor's card or ask them to spell their name. You should specifically ask what type of doctor they are. Knowing which group is in charge of decisions about your kidneys versus your heart issues will help you to know who to talk to for what problem.

Knowing when your doctor will be making rounds is important as well. Many doctors do hospital rounds early in the morning. Surgeons often start their operations early in the morning and perform them late into the evening. So, he or she may try to get patient rounds done before surgeries start. If you know the surgeon makes rounds every morning at 6 am, you can plan in advance to have someone with you then and to have your questions organized. If you don't ask them during that visit, it's unlikely that you'll see them again until the next day.

In addition to doctors' visits, you may also be taken from your room throughout the day to get a variety of tests. It's helpful to have a loved one keep track of what tests you're getting and ensure that you get the results of those tests communicated to you. You'd be surprised how many times patients get a variety of tests in the hospital and they have no idea what the tests are for or what their results are. You're paying for each one of these items and you're entitled to know what's being done and what the results are. You and your advocate also need to make sure that all the doctors involved in your care know what tests are being ordered for you.

TAKING NOTES AND MALPRACTICE CONCERNS

A word of caution about taking notes. Doctors are very concerned about malpractice issues, and a patient who takes copious notes can raise a red flag for them. Knowing that you want to have a good relationship with your doctor, make sure he or she understands that the reasons for the note-taking. Simply explaining that the notes help keep the family members who rotate in and out of your room coordinated should help to put your doctor's mind at ease. If you want to take pictures, you should explain why you are taking those pictures before doing so. For example, it may be helpful to refer to a picture of swelling in your feet when you talk to the primary care doctor you might not see for some time. These truthful explanations will help the doctor understand that you're not simply documenting your care so you can later sue him or her.

If for some reason you don't feel comfortable with the doctor and feel compelled to take pictures and notes to document care for a later lawsuit, it's best to change doctors immediately. Trust is one of the most important aspects of the doctor-patient relationship. Also patients need to have realistic expectations. Some individuals believe that healthcare providers have a magic wand and can fix any problem by merely putting a patient in the hospital, but this is rarely the case. If you've smoked for thirty years, are obese, or have never exercised, you'll likely have health conditions that aren't going to be solved by a single visit to the hospital.

How Do I Eat?

Meals in a hospital are often an important part of the day. For a patient, the days are very long, and meals offer a way to break up the day and have something to look forward to. Each hospital has a different way of managing patient meals. Old-fashioned hospitals simply deliver a pre-determined meal to your room. In most updated hospitals, you will have a menu to choose from and an ability to order your meals ahead of time.

Also remember that you may have some restrictions based on your illness as to what types of food you can eat. For instance, you may have a low sodium diet or a heart-healthy diet. The kitchen should know what your restrictions are, but, if for some reason, you call the kitchen and they allow you to order something that you aren't supposed to eat, make sure you inform them of your restrictions. Those restrictions are placed on you to help you get better.

If you're very sick, it's nice to have your family member order your meals for the day ahead of time. They can call the kitchen and order those items that you would like from the menu. You should not expect these meals to be "restaurant" grade quality; however, many hospitals have very good food.

If someone is staying with you in the room, you should be sensitive to the fact that your visitor may not be able to eat with you in the room. If you're in the ICU, there will be a limit on how many visitors you can have and it's unlikely that there can food in the room other than yours. This is for the health and safety of all patients and you should respect the hospital's rules. After all, you aren't there to visit with your friends but rather get well and go home.

Watch for Germs

Not surprisingly, hospitals have lots of germs. Although the hospital will do everything possible to prevent you from getting the illnesses of other patients, it's important that you do your part. You should not have any visitors who are sick and let family and friends know to keep small children at home. It's often helpful to keep alcohol wipes with you to sanitize anything that might be brought into the room. Also, your visitors should always wash their hands when they come into the room. Remember you're sick. That means that your immunity is low and your body is trying to fight off the illness. The last thing you want to do when in the hospital is to get sicker due to the people around you.

SHIFT CHANGE

Nurses work a certain amount of hours, known as a shift. Depending on which area of the hospital you are in and the various employees needed throughout the hospital, a nurse will only care for you over certain period of time. In most hospitals, when a shift starts, the nurse will write his or her name on a board in your room, so you can remember who they are for the time they are there. When the nurse goes off shift, they will give a "report" to the next nurse. During the "report," it will be very difficult for you to get much care unless you have an emergency. Therefore, you should make any requests you have prior to the shift change, and then repeat those requests to the new nurse when you first see him or her.

BE FRIENDLY AND COOPERATIVE WHENEVER POSSIBLE

Healthcare providers have a very difficult job. They have many demands on them and rarely have enough time with each of their patients. Generally, their days are very long and filled with stressful problems. You may have a friendly nurse one day and an unpleasant nurse the next. Your doctor may be lovely or may be a person who cannot communicate with a cockroach. No matter whether your healthcare provider is pleasant or not, it's very important for you to be friendly and cooperative. You know the saying: "you get more bees with honey." This is true in every part of the healthcare system.

If you're pleasant and can occasionally overlook a healthcare provider who's having a bad day, you will reap the rewards of receiving better care. No one wants to take care of a patient who's always unpleasant. Remember, you aren't in a hotel where the staff is hired to meet your every need. Every healthcare provider has many patients with different needs and you're just one of them. Try as best you can to do those things for yourself when you can. If your television isn't working, it's not a healthcare crisis. On the other hand, if you feel as though your doctor is constantly unpleasant and unwilling to communicate with you, it may be time to look for a new doctor.

THE BOTTOM LINE...

- Know that transferring to a different hospital is rarely an option.

- If you're at a hospital where your primary care physician is credentialed, ask him or her for specialist recommendations.

- Consider if a private room is a better option for you.

- Have someone with you whenever possible.

- If you're being treated by multiple specialists, designate one to coordinate your care with the others.

- Take notes (or have your visitors take them) so you have a clear record of your treatment, tests, and diagnosis.

- Don't expect restaurant-quality meals from a hospital.

- Do your part to keep from getting further infections and make sure your visitors do the same.

- Ask for anything you need prior to the nursing staff changing shifts.

- Be friendly and cooperative whenever possible.

7.

AVOID GETTING SICK IN THE FIRST PLACE

It should go without saying that you should do everything possible to avoid getting sick in the first place. Many people forget this basic rule. It's easy to stop exercising, gain weight, smoke, drink too much alcohol, miss sleep, and overdose on stress. Many doctors and nurses themselves have forgotten this basic rule.

So on to the "no brainer" advice that seems so hard to follow.

TAKE CARE OF YOURSELF

Remember, an "ounce prevention is worth a pound of care." Neglecting your health and then expecting the healthcare industry to fix the problems that you spent years creating is not a good recipe for success. You can go into any cardiac wing at a hospital and ask any of the patients whether they wish they had taken care of their health prior to their heart attack and you will get a resounding "yes." It's never too late to start.

Also, remember to take simple precautions daily to remain well. Start with washing your hands. Never touch your nose, mouth, or eyes without washing your hands. You're in contact with germs wherever you go. Hand washing is a simple tool to keep well. Try to not to share food or beverages with others. This is a simple skill to teach your children in school. Not sharing a chocolate milk carton with your friend might help prevent a cold.

Remember to cover your mouth with a tissue when you cough or sneeze. Dispose of the tissue yourself. These may seem like silly suggestions but avoiding germs is the best way to protect against common illnesses that can, in turn, lead to more serious issues. Stay hydrated and get plenty of rest if you want to keep from getting sick. Eating healthy foods will also help keep you from getting sick.

GET REGULAR CHECK-UPS

Make sure to see your doctor on a regular basis. The **Affordable Care Act** (otherwise known as "ObamaCare") now makes healthcare mandatory and available to everyone. Make sure you sign up for health insurance. Although we complain about the cost of healthcare insurance, we forget how much we spend each month on our own bad health habits. If we cut out the cigarettes and alcohol, the savings would more than cover the cost of health insurance.

Be certain to avoid people who have colds or the flu if possible. Get regular vaccinations. This is especially true as you age. Many seniors die from pneumonia that they contract after a cold or the flu.

HAVE GOOD RELATIONSHIPS WITH OTHERS

Another important factor in maintaining your health is keeping good relationships with those around you. Many scientific studies have proven time and time again that those individuals with a positive attitude and strong relationships are healthier than those people who tend to keep to themselves. You should strive to wake up every morning being grateful for the day ahead. Take a walk, eat a healthy breakfast, and remind yourself how lucky you are to not be sick.

THE BOTTOM LINE...

- Avoid getting sick in the first place by acting on the "no-brainer" advice everyone finds so hard to follow.

- Take simple precautions like washing your hands regularly and not sharing food and drink.

- Get regular checkups and take advantage of preventive care, including health screenings such as mammograms and colonoscopies.

- Have good relationships with others. Engaging with those around you and keeping a positive attitude play a significant role in keeping you well.

CONCLUSION

Knowing what to do when you get sick is an important skill to have. Being proactive regarding your health is always the best option. Waiting until you get sick is often too late. Talk to your family about each other's health needs. Make sure you know how you're feeling and call the doctor before your condition becomes more serious. If you have a life-threatening illness, don't hesitate to call 911. But for other, non-threatening illnesses and injuries, use common sense, a little planning, and a little "triage" to avoid a lot of unnecessary time and expense. And remember, staying healthy is the best way to avoid getting sick altogether.

TERMS TO KNOW

Affordable Care Act: Federal law signed by President Barack Obama in 2010 that fundamentally reformed the U.S. healthcare system and the health insurance industry.

Co-pay: Flat fee an individual pays as an "out of pocket" expense when he or she visits the doctor.

Credentialed: Term referring to a physician's ability to practice medicine at a given hospital. Administrators will regularly review a physician's training, practice history, and certifications among other factors to determine if he or she may practice at their hospital.

Deductible: The amount an individual must spend before a health insurance plan will make payments for your healthcare. Some services, for example preventative care, are exempt from the deductible.

Intern: Physician in training who has not yet graduated from medical school.

Medicare: Insurance program run by the federal government that provides health coverage to people over the age of sixty-five. Medicare also provides coverage for people with certain disabilities as well as those with end stage renal disease.

Observation: Status determined by a hospital that means a patient in the emergency room is too sick to go home, but not sick enough to be admitted to the hospital. Patients under observation may have tests run or be monitored to see if further symptoms develop.

On call: Status in which a physician is ready to respond when needed to care for patients.

Patient advocate office: Department at a hospital that represents patient needs to administrators while assisting patients in resolving individual concerns.

Preventative care: Medical procedures and practices, such as annual physicals and health screenings such as colonoscopies and mammograms, that aid in keeping a patient healthy by identifying serious illnesses early and promoting good habits.

Resident: Physician in training who has graduated from medical school and is learning his or her specialty.

Triage: Method by which healthcare professionals prioritize which patients should be treated first based upon the relative severity and urgency of the patient's condition.

Urgent care facility: A medical facility that provides treatment for non-emergency illnesses and injuries when an individual cannot see his or her primary care physician.

LORI-ANN'S ON YOUR SIDE

"When I need health care advice I can understand and
follow, I call Lori-Ann. She knows her stuff!"
M. Diane Vogt, JD

"Lori-Ann is my "go-to" expert on healthcare law.
She makes it understandable and easy to follow
for our doctors and their patients, too."
Michele Nichols, The Physician Alliance

"Lori-Ann knows the healthcare system inside and out. Whenever
we have questions about healthcare, Lori-Ann has the answers."
Mike Gerstenlauer, St. John-Macomb Hospital

"Whenever my family has a health care issue, Lori-
Ann is my first call for the best advice."
Donna Curran

"Getting coverage for prescription drugs can be a big problem for
patients. Lori-Ann knows the insider secrets to making it easy."
Coreen Buehrer

"Lori-Ann has also lived the difficult issues that families confront on
a daily basis as they struggle with the bewildering maze of hospitals,
multiple specialists and insurance companies as our family's tire-
less advocate for our father. No mother grizzly ever fought for her
cubs with more passion than Lori-Ann looked out for our dad."
Stephen Rickard, J.D., MPA

ABOUT THE AUTHOR

Lori-Ann Rickard is one of the country's top healthcare lawyers. For over three decades, she has advised leading hospitals, doctors, laboratories, and other healthcare providers. Now she offers her expertise to patients and their families through the Easy Healthcare Series from HealthSpin.

Lori-Ann is also a single mom of two beautiful daughters. One of her daughters was very sick when she was born. Already caring for a toddler and managing a developing career, Lori-Ann used her professional experience to create quick, effective strategies to make the healthcare system work for her as she sought the best treatment possible for her sick baby. Later, Lori-Ann served as the primary caregiver and medical coordinator for her proud, independent parents when they became unable to care for themselves. Through their wellness challenges, her daughter's illness, and in helping friends over the past thirty years, Lori-Ann has used her unique position in the industry to create easy healthcare solutions that work for everyone around her. These solutions will work for you and your family, too.

Lori-Ann Rickard is a healthcare insider who knows what it means to be a patient and a caregiver. The Easy Healthcare Series brings you the benefit of Lori-Ann Rickard's expertise. Let her show you how you can Spin Your Healthcare Your Way.

MORE BY LORI-ANN RICKARD

Visit myhealthspin.com to download your free copy
of *Easy Healthcare: What You Need First!*
ALSO AVAILABLE FROM HEALTHSPIN:

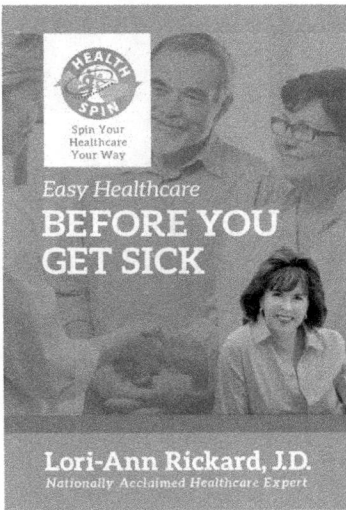

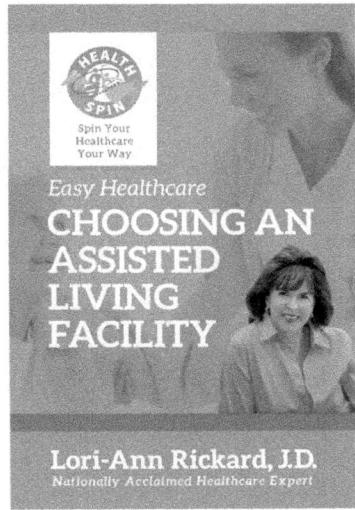

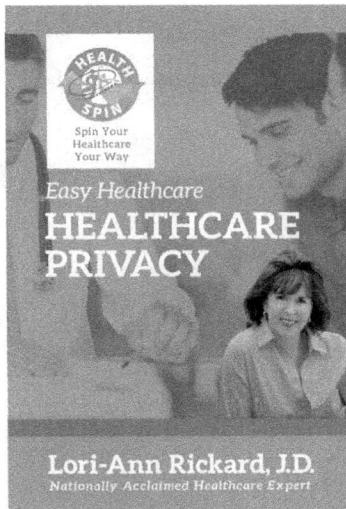

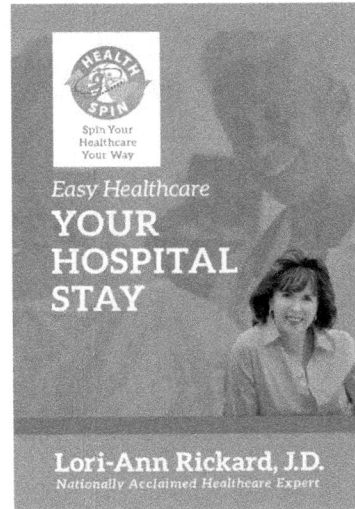

* 9 7 8 1 9 4 0 7 6 7 0 9 3 *